Rapid Weight Loss Hypnosis For Beginners

A Superlative Guide To Guided Meditations, Affirmations& Hypnosis To Help You Develop Self Love, Confidence, Mindfulness, And Healthy Eating Habits

Written By

Melissa Greger

Table of Contents

INTRODUCTION

Thank you for purchasing this book!

Large or overweight kids may confront long stretches of battle with their relationship to food and mental self-portrait issues. Hypnotherapy could be an early mediation to address the issue of youth stoutness. These are on the whole individuals who may well significantly profit by the effective treatment of Hypnosis.

Enjoy your reading!

Gastric Band Hypnotherapy

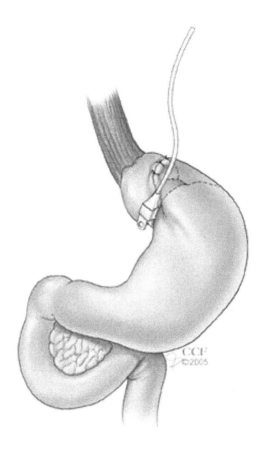

Propose to the subliminal that you've had a gastric band fitted around your stomach to help you get more fit. Thought about a final retreat, gastric band medical procedure includes installing a group around the top piece of the stomach. This restricts the measure of food you can honestly eat, empowering weight loss. It's a surgery, and along these lines accompanies expected dangers and complexities. The method utilized by trance inducers to get the inner mind to confine the measure of food an individual can genuinely eat, making them feel full after eating next to the hotel in the wake of attempting different strategies Gastric band trance can be utilized to assist individuals with getting thinner, without the dangers that accompany the medical procedure. Numerous subliminal specialists use a two-dimensional methodology. First, they hope to recognize the underlying driver of your enthusiastic eating. Utilizing entrancing, the advisor can urge you to recollect since quite a while ago overlooked encounters encompassing food that might be subliminally influencing you now. Tending to and perceiving any undesirable idea designs containing food can be useful before doing gastric band hypnotherapy.

Next, the subliminal specialist will do the virtual gastric band treatment. The methodology is intended to propose, at an inner mind causing you to Trance specialist Becca Tears clarifies why diets don't work for weight loss: Diets don't in general arrangement with the lasting way of life changes required, for example, a possible long haul change in our dietary patterns and demeanor to food. Many eating routine plans are impermanent and can be hard to keep up on an ongoing premise, frequently because they are excessively prohibitive or they thoroughly deny us of our preferred nourishments. These systems can be clung to the present moment; however, don't work so well over the long haul. By making us tally calories or deliberately measure partition size or even absolutely exclude kinds of nourishments, numerous weight control plans can make us increasingly fixated on food and our eating. This can remove the joy from eating and can lead us to long for a more considerable amount of specific nourishments, and an eating regimen gorge/gorge cycle can begin.

How Gastric Band Trance Functions

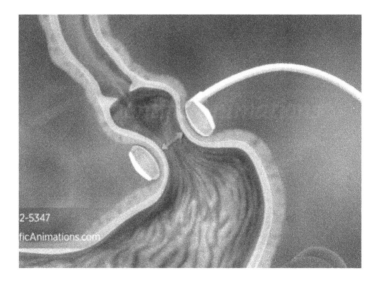

Utilizing unwinding strategies, a trance inducer will place you into a condition of mesmerizing. In this casual express, your inner mind is increasingly open to the proposal. Now subliminal specialists make recommendations to your psyche. With gastric band hypnotherapy, this proposal is that you've had a physical band fitted. The ego is incredible, so in case you're subliminal acknowledges these recommendations, your conduct will change in like manner. Proposals encompassing certainty and oversight will be made to assist you with focusing on this adjustment in the way of life. Numerous specialists will likewise show self-entrancing procedures to improve the work you've done after the meeting. Teaching yourself on sustenance and exercise is regularly advised, too, to advance physical health and prosperity.

Right, and sensitive alteration of the band is fundamental for weight decrease and the drawn-out achievement of the method. Changes (furthermore called "fills") may be performed using an X-bar fluoroscope with the objective that the radiologist can study the circumstance of the band, the port, and the tubing that runs between the port and the gathering. The patient is given a little cup of liquid containing an undeniable or white radio-cloudy fluid-like barium. When swallowed, the fluid clearly shows up on the X bar, and it looked as it goes down the throat and through the restriction realized by the band. The radiologist is then prepared to see the level of limitation in the gathering and to overview if there are potential or making issues of concern. These may fuse extending of the throat, and increased pocket, prolapsed stomach (when part of the stomach moves into the band where it doesn't have a spot), breaking down, or migration. Reflux type reactions may show too exceptional a constraint, and further examination may be required.

Under specific conditions, the fluid is removed from the band before further assessment and re-evaluation. In various cases, new clinical methods may be required (for instance, departure of the gathering) should gastric breaking down or relative trouble be recognized. Some prosperity specialists adjust the band without the usage of X-shaft control (fluoroscopy). In these cases, the pro assesses the patient's weight decrease and potential reflex symptoms depicted by the patient, for instance, indigestion, regurgitating forward, or chest torment. From this information, the pro picks whether a band change is necessary. Changes are consistently determined whether a patient has raga.

Standard-Fill Change

Standard-fill change will routinely find they will contribute more vitality talking about the adjustment and their progression than the proper fill itself, which all things considered will take just around one to two minutes. In any case, for fulfilled patients, this kind of plenty is past the domain of creative mind, given issues such as midway upset of the port, or excess tissue over the port creation it challenging to choose its particular region. In these cases, a fluoroscope will, generally, be used. It is an undeniably fundamental practice for the band not to be filled at the clinical system, but a couple of pros choose to place a modest amount in the gathering at the hour of clinical method. The stomach will, by and large, swell after a clinical methodology, and it is possible that too phenomenal a restriction would be practiced at whatever point involved around at that point. Various prosperity authorities make the main change someplace in the scope of 4 and a month and a half postoperatively to allow the stomach time to patch. Starting now and into the foreseeable future, fills continue changing. No exact number of changes required can be given. The proportion of the saline/isotonic plan needed for the band varies from patient to comprehension. There are barely any people who find they needn't waste time with a fill at all and have sufficient restrictions rapidly following clinical methods. Others may require important acclimations to the best the band can hold.

<u>The Method</u>

The conference where you talk about what you would like to pick up. The methodology itself is intended to imitate gastric band medical procedure, to enable your inner mind to trust it has genuinely occurred. To make the experience progressively valid, numerous trance specialists will fuse the sounds and scents of a working theater. Your specialist will start by bringing you into a profoundly loosened up state, otherwise called a trance. Upgrade the experience, to convince your subliminal that what's being said is truly transpiring. As recently referenced, different recommendations might be joined during the method to expand fearlessness. When the process is finished, your subliminal specialist may show you some self-entrancing strategies to assist you with remaining on target at home. Some trance specialists will demand that you return for follow-up arrangements to screen the virtual band's prosperity and to make any changes. Meetings as a significant aspect of a drawn-out weight the board plan. This permits the trance inducer to work with you to address fundamental issues encompassing food and confidence. The brain is frequently best for those looking for weight loss.

By What Means Will I Feel After?

The general point of gastric band mesmerizing is to empower a more beneficial connection with food. At the point when your inner mind trusts you have had a gastric band fitted, it will accept your stomach is littler. This, thus, causes your cerebrum to convey messages that you are full in the wake of expending less food. The system ought to be a lovely and loosening up understanding, with many people announcing a sentiment of quiet when they come out of a trance.

Will It Work for Me?

A typical inquiry for that difficult Hypnotherapy just because is - will it work for me? Shockingly is anything but a primary instance of yes or no; it is, to a great extent, up to you. Hypnotherapy helps individuals with a scope of concerns; however, it is especially valuable with regards to evolving propensities. Consequently, it is frequently fruitful in assisting individuals in creating good dieting propensities and shed pounds. Weight loss framework, it will require your absolute duty. You are bound to get what you need from gastric band hypnotherapy on the off chance that you put stock all the while and your specialist. Being agreeable and believing your trance specialist is fundamental. This is the reason it is prompted that you set aside some effort to explore trance inducers in your general vicinity and discover progressively about them, how they work, and what their capabilities involve. You can organize to meet with them before the method to guarantee you feel good with them. If you are focused on making a way of life change, have faith in the strategy, and trust your trance inducer, gastric band trance should work for you. This doesn't occur without a doubt, just in your psyche mind. Your brain, at that point, trusts you have a gastric band fitted where you imagine implies you eat increasingly slow less, as you intellectually feel a lot fuller a lot faster. Your craving is radically decreased, and weight loss is undeniably increasingly common given the gastric band trance meetings. It's a sheltered and a profoundly viable technique for weight loss and appeared all through clinical preliminaries worldwide and is regularly alluded to as the Hypnos band.

The Trancelike Rest

Hypnosis regularly includes a prologue to the strategy during which the subject is informed that proposals for innovative encounters will be introduced. The trancelike enlistment is an all-encompassing starting proposal for utilizing one's creative mind and may contain further elaborations of the presentation. A sleep-inducing system is used to urge and assess reactions to proposals. When utilizing Hypnosis, one individual (the subject) is guided by another (the trance inducer) to react to recommendations for changes in abstract understanding, adjustments in perception, sensation, feeling, thought or conduct. People can likewise learn self-hypnosis, which is the demonstration of overseeing trancelike techniques all alone. On the off chance that the subject reacts to trancelike proposals, it is, for the most part, derived that Hypnosis has been initiated. Many accept that mesmerizing reactions and encounters are typical for a trancelike state. While some believe that it isn't essential to utilize "hypnosis" as a feature of the entrancing acceptance, others see it as fundamental.

Intriguing Ongoing Weight Loss Posts from Moose and Doc

- 6 Top Tips to Quick Weight loss

- Weight Misfortune Inspirations

- Lose Weight Quick and stage plan on the most proficient method to

- Lose Weight in seven days without counting calories

- How to lose gut fat Quick

- Green Tea Weight loss: Certainty or Fiction?

- Learn how to lose Face Fat Quick

Fascinating Ongoing Eating Routine Posts from Moose and Doc

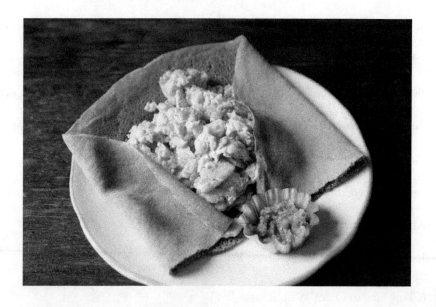

- The Mediterranean Eating routine

- The Run Diet

- The Atkins Diet Returned to

- The H.C.G.H.C.G. Diet

- The Paleo Diet

- Stop Dreaming and begin shedding with the Dukan Diet.

- Military Franticness! The multi-day Military Eating routine Arrangement

Story Hypnosis

Story Telling Hypnosis, utilization of storytelling in Hypnotherapy. Stories and anecdotes are precious in Hypnotherapy. Individuals usually are used to turning out to be put resources into accounts, regardless of whether read or performed on T.V.T.V. or big screen. For thousands of years, exhibitions and

stories have been utilized to pass on the importance and to send messages to the crowd.

Utilizing Stories During Hypnotherapy

In a condition of Hypnosis, which is the casual state utilized in Hypnotherapy, accounts can be used to delineate issues, depict a change, or give another inclination or point of view on a circumstance or problem. Now and again, re-surrounding the question as though it is something looked by a more unusual makes an extraordinary disposition create. Here and there, re- encircling makes the individual acknowledge they can handle something that was excessively terrifying or appeared to enormous an issue to defeat beforehand.

Utilizing Story Stories in Hypnotherapy

In some cases, the story can be symbolic and not exacting. Discussing a creature, tree, or rock may appear odd, yet the portrayal can be symbolic and indeed allude to the customer. For instance, considering a tall stable tree may think about the individual's shrouded qualities, a profound unadulterated pool of water may be the beginning of a depiction welcoming further close to home reflection. Nearly anything can be utilized justified and fitting conditions to draw correlations and tell a remedial story.

Hypnotherapy for Individual Change

Storytelling is frequently utilized in the kind of Hypnotherapy that identifies with personal transformation. It opens the possibility of another account, another unique story that could create. That story could identify with

expanded certainty, more grounded own confidence, inspiration, or an all the more mindful demeanor to oneself or others.

Styles of Hypnotherapy

Milton Erickson broadly utilized stories a great deal in both express structure hypnotherapy meetings and modified state work, where he didn't seem to "mesmerize" the customer, yet rather necessarily reveal to them a story. Different advisors have utilized stories with more youthful customers, and Sideris is a model of Hypnotherapy explicitly using story and account.

Supporting Hypnotherapy with Analysis and

Psychotherapy

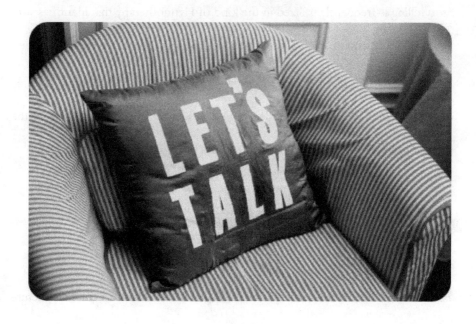

Story creation depends on a complete comprehension of the customer's circumstance. The story must be symbolic, dependent on data accumulated. Accordingly, analysis, psychotherapy, directing, or other talking treatments are typically used to increase an image of the present circumstance, from which to structure a "change" story. Stuart prepared in therapy and Hypnotherapy from 1993-1996 (remotely NVQ authorize and surveyed recognition course and C.N.H.C. accreditation course using S.S.M.S.S.M.), being evaluated on more than 200 customers (more than 1,000 customer hours) with a necessary positive input pace of 80%. From that point forward, he has contemplated different types of psychotherapy and advising and has finished C.P.D.C.P.D. (nonstop professional turn of events) in the scope of zones, including Sidereus narrating. Different zones remembered eastern brain research projects and contemplation and an MSc for Brain research. Stuart is a

C.N.H.C. enlisted trance specialist. C.N.H.C. is the willful controller for corresponding treatments set up with U.K.U.K. Government financing and Backing. It is likewise an A.R.A.R. conspire. The Professional Norms Expert directs licensed Registers for human services specialists not expose to the legal guideline. Stuart is also enrolled in the FHT AR plot. Stuart rehearses in Edinburgh, Falkirk, Dublin, and Glasgow.Catchphrases

Hypnotherapy, Hypnosis, Daze, Self-Hypnosis, Anecdote, Narrating, account, treatment, change process, perception, reflection, psychotherapy, analysis, directing, Edinburgh, Glasgow, Falkirk, psychoanalyst, psychotherapist, instructor, trance specialist, trance inducer, M.C.B.T., C.B.T.C.B.T., C.B.A.C.B.A., I.P.T.I.P.T., N.L.PN.L.P

History of Hypnosis

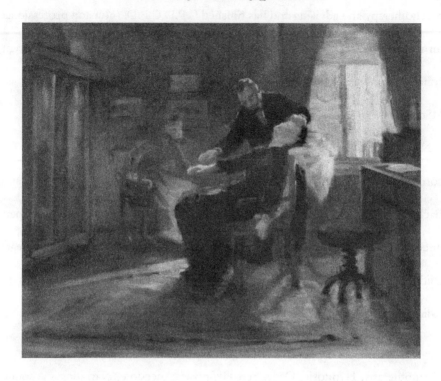

Harry Arons was the greatest benefactor in the 20th century to the acknowledgment of Hypnosis by the clinical and psychological health network with his practically month to month instructional classes around the U.S. U.S. for more than five decades. During his 52-year career, he prepared a considerable number of specialists, therapists, and specialists in the use of Hypnosis to support their patients. He likewise spearheaded in using Hypnosis in the criminal examination and worked effectively with notable lawyers like F. Lee Bailey in the well-known Coppolino murder preliminary. His hypnosis strategies and techniques are still broadly utilized by professionals right up 'til the present time. The improvement of ideas, convictions, and practices identified with Hypnosis and Hypnotherapy has been archived since ancient to present-day times. Albeit often seen as one nonstop history, the term hypnosis was authored during the 1880s in France, which was somewhere in the range of twenty years after the passing of James Plait, who had embraced the term sleep induction in 1841. Mesh embraced the term subliminal therapy (which explicitly applied to the condition of the subject, as opposed to methods used by the administrator) to differentiate his own, one of a kind.

20th-Century Subliminal Therapy

Emile Coue

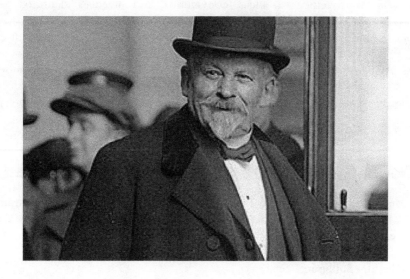

Emile Coue (1857 1926), a French drug specialist and, as indicated by Charles Baudouin, the author concentrated with Liebeault in 1885 and 1886, disposed of the 'hypnosis' of Bernheim and Liebeault (c. 1886), received the 'tranceliketrancelike influence' of Mesh (c. 1901) and made what got known as the (la methode Coue), focused on the advancement of conscious autosuggestion. His strategy was an arranged grouping of discerning, efficient, complicatedly built, subject-focused hypnotherapeutic associations that concentrate on the essentialness of both oblivious and cognizant autosuggestion, conveyed an assortment of very much cleaned useful judgment clarifications, an influential arrangement of experiential activities, an intensely strong trance induction focused conscience reinforcing intercession and, at last, point by point guidance in the particular ceremony through which his experimentally decided recipe "Consistently, all around, I'm showing signs of improvement and better" was to act naturally regulated twice every day. A significant part of crafted by mid-20th-century self-improvement educators (for example, for example, Norman Vincent Peale, Robert H. Schuller, and

W. Merciful Stone) was gotten from that of Coue. Boris Sidis

Boris Sidis (1867 1923), a Ukraine-brought into the world American analyst and therapist concentrating under William James at Harvard College, figured this law of recommendation: Suggestibility fluctuates as the measure of disaggregation, and contrarily as the unification of cognizance. Disaggregation

alludes to the split between the ordinary waking awareness and the inner mind.

Johannes Schultz

The German therapist Johannes Schultz adjusted the speculations of Abbe Faria and Emile Coué and recognizing sure equals to methods in yoga and contemplation. He called his arrangement of self-hypnosis Autogenic preparing.

Gustave Le Bon

Gustave Le Bon's investigation of group brain science looked at the impacts of a pioneer of a gathering to Hypnosis. Le Bon utilized the suggestibility idea.

Sigmund Freud

Hypnosis, which toward the finish of the nineteenth century had become a famous marvel, precisely because of Charcot's open sleep induction meetings, was essential in the innovation of analysis by Sigmund Freud, an understudy of Charcot. Freud later saw a few of the examinations of Liébeault and Hippolyte Bernheim in Nancy. Back in Vienna, he created abreaction treatment utilizing Hypnosis with Josef Breuer. When Sigmund Freud limited its utilization in psychiatry, in the first half of the only remaining century, subliminal stage specialists kept it alive more than doctors.

Platonov and Pavlov

Russian medication has had broad involvement in obstetric Hypnosis. Platonov, during the 1920s, turned out to be notable for his Hypno-obstetric victories. Dazzled by this methodology, Stalin later set up an across the country program headed by Velvoski, who initially consolidated hypnosis with Pavlov's procedures, yet in the end, utilized the last solely. Having visited Russia, Fernand Lamaze took back to France "labor without torment through the mental strategy," which indicated more reflexology than sleep-inducing motivation.

20th-Century Wars

Hypnosis in the treatment of despondencies prospered during World War I, World War II, and the Korean War. Hypnosis methods were converged with psychiatry and were particularly helpful in the treatment of what is referred to today as Post Awful Pressure Disorder.

William McDougall

William McDougall (1871 1944), an English therapist, rewarded warriors with "shell stun" and censured certain parts of the Freudian hypothesis, for example, the idea of abreaction.

Clark L. Structure

The cutting edge investigation of sleep induction is generally considered to have started during the 1920s with Clark Leonard Body (1884 1952) at Yale College. A test therapist, his work Hypnosis and Suggestibility (1933) was a thorough investigation of the marvel, utilizing measurable and test examination. Body's studies earnestly showed for the last time that Hypnosis had no association with rest ("Hypnosis isn't rest, . it has no unique relationship to rest, and the entire.

The principle consequence of Structure's examination was to get control over the extreme cases of subliminal specialists, particularly concerning remarkable upgrades in comprehension or the faculties under Hypnosis. Structure's trials demonstrated the truth of some old-style wonders, for example, intellectually actuated torment decrease and evident hindrance of memory review. In any case, Clark's work clarified that these impacts could be accomplished without Hypnosis being viewed as a particular state, yet rather because of proposal and inspiration, which was a harbinger of the conduct way to deal with Hypnosis. Essentially, moderate increments in certain physical limits and changes to the edge of tactile incitement could be actuated mentally; lessening impacts could be particularly emotional.

Andrew Salter

During the 1940s, Andrew Salter (1914 1996) acquainted with American treatment the Pavlovian technique for negating, contradicting, and assaulting convictions. In the molded reflex, he has discovered what he saw as the quintessence of Hypnosis. He, in this way, gave a resurrection to tranceliketrancelike influence by consolidating it with old-style molding. Ivan Pavlov had himself prompted a modified state in pigeons, that he alluded to as

"Cortical Restraint," which some later scholars accept was some type of mesmerizing state.

English Sleep induction Act

In the Unified Realm, the Subliminal therapy Act 1952 was founded to control stage trance specialists' open stimulations.

English Clinical Affiliation, 1955

On 23 April 1955, the English Clinical Affiliation (B.M.A.B.M.A.) affirmed the utilization of Hypnosis in the territories of psychoneuroses and hypoaesthesia in torment the executives in labor and medical procedure. As of now, the B.M.A.B.M.A. likewise prompted all doctors and clinical understudies to get the principal preparing in Hypnosis.

1956, Pope's endorsement of Hypnosis. The Roman Catholic Church restricted subliminal therapy until the mid-20th century when, in 1956, Pope Pius XII gave his endorsement of Hypnosis. He expressed that the utilization of Hypnosis by medicinal services professionals for conclusion and treatment is allowed. In a location from the Vatican on Hypnosis in labor, the Pope gave these rules:

Subliminal therapy is a genuine issue, and not something to fiddle with. In its logical use, the precautionary measures directed by both science and decent quality must be followed. Under the part of sedation, it is administered by the same standards from different types of sedation.

American Clinical Affiliation, 1958

In 1958, the American Clinical Affiliation endorsed a report on the clinical employments of Hypnosis. It empowered research on Hypnosis even though bringing up that a few parts of Hypnosis are obscure and questionable. Be that as it may, in June 1987, the A.M.A.' sA.M.A.'s strategy-making body canceled all A.M.A.A.M.A. strategies from 1881 1958 (other than two not identifying with Hypnosis).

American Mental Affiliation

Two years after A.M.A.A.M.A. endorsement, the American Mental Affiliation embraced Hypnosis as a part of psychology.

Ernest Hilgard and others

Studies proceeded after the Subsequent Universal War. Hairdresser, Hilgard, Orne, and Sarbin likewise created significant examination made the Stanford scales, a normalized scale for helplessness to Hypnosis, and appropriately inspected defenselessness across age-gatherings and sex. Hilgard proceeded to examine tangible duplicity (1965) and incited sedation and absence of pain (1975).

<u>Harry Arons (1914-1997)</u>

Harry Arons was the greatest supporter in the twentieth century to the acknowledgment of Hypnosis by the clinical and emotional health network with his practically month to month instructional classes around the U.S. U.S. for more than five decades. During his 52-year vocation, he prepared a considerable number of specialists, psychologists, and psychiatrists in the utilization of Hypnosis to support their patients. He additionally spearheaded in using Hypnosis in the criminal examination and worked effectively with notable lawyers like F. Lee Bailey in the acclaimed Coppolino murder preliminary. His hypnosis methods and techniques are still broadly utilized by experts to this day.

Dave Elman

Dave Elman (1900 1967) assisted with advancing the clinical utilization of Hypnosis from 1949 until his cardiovascular failure in 1962. Elman's meaning of Hypnosis is as yet utilized today by skilled hypnotherapists. Even though Elman had no clinical preparation, Gil Boyne (a significant instructor of Hypnosis) over and again expressed that Dave Elman prepared more doctors and dentists in the utilization of hypnotism than any other individual in the U.SU.S.

Dave Elman is likewise known for acquainting quick enlistments with the field of hypnotism. An enlistment strategy he presented more than fifty years back is as yet one of the supported acceptances utilized by numerous individuals of the present specialists. He set incredible WeightWeight on what he called "the Esdaile state" or the "sleep-inducing extreme lethargies," which, as indicated by Elman, had not been purposely instigated since Scottish specialist James Esdaile last accomplished it. This was a lamentable and historically mistaken decision of wording on Elman's part. Esdaile never utilized what we currently call Hypnosis even on a single event; he used something freely looking like mesmerism (otherwise called creature magnetism).

Ormond McGill

Ormond McGill (1913 2005), phase hypnotist and Hypnotherapist, was the "Senior member of American Hypnotists" and essayist of the fundamental "Reference book of Real Stage Hypnotism" (1947).

U.S. U.S. Definition For, Hypnotherapist

The U.S. U.S. (Division of Work) Index of Word related Titles accompanying description:

Talks with customers to decide the idea of the issue. Gets ready customers to enter trancelike states by clarifying how hypnosis functions and what customers will understand enthusiastic suggestibility. Instigates sleep-inducing state in customers utilizing individualized strategies and methods of Hypnosis dependent on an understanding of test outcomes and analysis of customer's concern. May prepare customer in self-hypnosis molding. A few states hold the expression "Therapist" to be authorized, clinical experts. Along these lines, utilizing this term and not being an authorized proficient would rehearse without a permit.

U.K.U.K. National Word related Gauges

National Word connected Gauges (N.O.S.N.O.S.) for Hypnotherapy was published in 2002 by Abilities for Health, the Administration's Part Aptitudes Board for the U.K.U.K. health industry. The Capabilities and Educational program Authority began presenting discretionary declarations and confirmations at a global level through National Granting Bodies by surveying learning results of preparing/authorizing earlier experiential learning.

Hypnosis to Avoid Binge and Emotional Eating

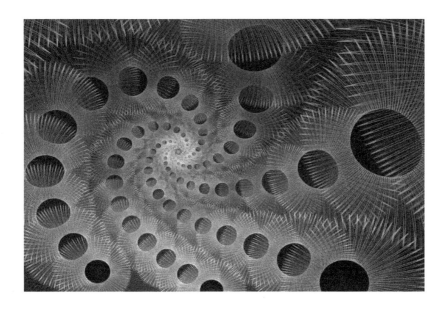

In this way, if you've been abstaining from excessive food intake and practicing yet are continually focused on, you probably won't address the difficulty of keeping the weight on. Once more, stress discharges hormones that store additional fat precisely what we don't need! This can even fuel a pattern of pressure: You can't get more fit since you're focused on, which makes you worried about not having the option to get more fit. It's a simple example to stall out; however, you can break it — and reflection can help.

To all the more likely arrangement with a push or kill it, you must initially comprehend what causes most of it in your life. A few stressors are anything but difficult to recognize; however, others can be increasingly unpretentious. The Well Be is an armband that capacities to some degree like a physical action tracker, yet it's the first of its sort to concentrate on enthusiastic health. Bilstein includes, "It even reveals to you who and what exercises throughout your life trigger passionate pressure, and in this manner can assist you with concocting elective ways of dealing with stress that may aid weight loss." See the Well Be in real life in the video underneath with Bilstein and editorial manager Linda Rodgers:

Indian limitation

The Ministry of Health and Family Government assistance, Administration wholly expressed that Hypnotherapy is a suggested method of treatment in India, to be rehearsed uniquely by the properly prepared workforce.

What Is Hypnotherapy?

To comprehend the distinction between Hypnosis and Hypnotherapy, consider Hypnosis an instrument and Hypnotherapy as the utilization of an apparatus. In S.A.T.S.A.T. terms, Hypnotherapy is to hypnotism as artistry treatment is to craftsmanship.

- The meaning of Hypnotherapy is evident from the word itself. Hypnotherapy is the act of Hypnosis for medicinal purposes.

- As it were, on the off chance that you are an expert emotional health therapist or clinical specialist and you're utilizing Hypnosis to enable a customer to defeat a psychological or state of being, you're rehearsing Hypnotherapy.

- The mesmerizing daze state is an astoundingly versatile device for taking care of mental and physical medical issues. Here are only a couple of ways emotional wellness and clinical experts use Hypnotherapy:

- v Helping individuals quit smoking or decrease gorging by centering their brains and recommending more advantageous conduct.

- v Accessing the brain-body connect to diminish interminable and intense torment, including during medical procedure and labor. Hypnotherapy has likewise demonstrated viable against severe physical tribulations like crabby inside disorder and dermatological conditions.

- v Diving profound into the psyche brain reveals and treats the main drivers of psychological wellness issues, such as wretchedness, uneasiness, P.T.S.D., and dependence.

- We'll center the remainder of this article on that last use. The same number of hypnotherapists have discovered, the unconscious state is the way to opening the shrouded profundities of our brains, recollections, and inspirations.

- (You would be surprised how regularly Hypnotherapy is utilized in current

41

medication and psychotherapy. Realize why specialists and therapists are going to Hypnotherapy in our free whitepaper, "A definitive Manual for Clinical Hypnotherapy Procedures.")

How Accomplishes Hypnotherapy Work?

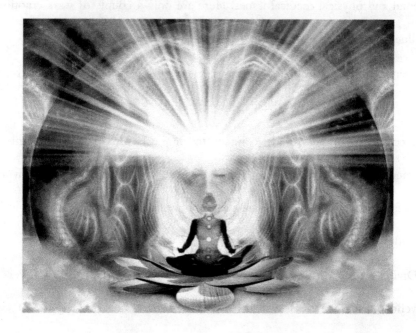

The most remarkable element of the unconscious state is how it associates our cognizant personalities to our psyche minds. Hypnotherapy master Diane Zimberoff, the prime supporter of the Health Establishment, thinks about the psyche brain to a P.C.' sP.C.'s record framework. Our inner mind resembles our hard drive: we store each understanding, feeling, and though we've had. In the loose, hyper-centered condition of Hypnosis — under the direction of a hypnotherapist — we can run a Google search on our inner mind, pulling up the curbed recollections and covered feelings at the base of our psychological health difficulties.Zimberoff expresses: "Each unfortunate current conduct, for example, smoking, losing one's temper, excessive liquor utilization, or impulsive indulging, has a chain of occasions that established the framework for the entirety of our current undesirable decisions. Through the 'memory chip' that has been set down in the psyche mind, we can follow back the encounters and subliminal decisions we made as youngsters that might be driving us to the conduct that is not, at this point, sound for us." This works out in a right way past primary suggestibility. Experienced hypnotherapist Judi Vitale portrays two different ways to deal with helping a customer quit smoking utilizing Hypnotherapy:

"With Hypnosis, you may assist somebody with halting smoking by recommending the taste or smell of cigarettes is more awful than it is. In any case, a hypnotherapist can likewise utilize age relapse to look at the drive that fills the customer's propensity and discovers old ends and practices. The mending will happen when the customer makes new decisions about old recollections and picks new practices as opposed to smoking." Because the subsequent methodology gets at the base of the issue, Vitale says, it is considerably more successful than the first. Results come rapidly, and they last.

Front line cerebrum imaging innovation currently gives us a window into the physical indications of Hypnotherapy. When they examined the minds of 57 people experiencing trance, Stanford scientists announced that areas of the cerebrum related to understanding and change demonstrated "adjusted action and network."(Hypnotherapy is a proof-based mental and physical health treatment method. Peruse the science with our free 140-page assemblage of trance and hypnotherapy references.)What Emotional health Issues Would Hypnotherapy be able to Help With? A considerable lot of the trance inducers prepared by the Health Establishment have seen Hypnotherapy as best against issues originating from quelled injury. Been frequenting them in a manner that appeared as if they were continually remembering that damaging second," Vitale says. Subliminal specialist Wendy Pugh discloses to us. Hypnotherapy works extraordinarily well when youth injury has happened. Present working," she says. For instance, Pugh says, numerous individuals don't understand how profoundly their current tensions are established in occasions of the past. By testing the past, covered feelings, and the bogus ends secured your customers' inner mind minds, you can utilize Hypnotherapy to treat the absolute generally crippling and tireless emotional health difficulties.

Hypnosis for Portion Control Sessions

Reflection is mainly the demonstration of concentrating on turning out to be increasingly careful. The American Reflection Society clarifies that "during contemplation, the consideration streams internally as opposed to taking part in the outside universe of action." As indicated by the association, a contemplation practice can stir positive characteristics in you. Nutrition should be varied and meet the requirements for proteins, fats, carbohydrates, vitamins, minerals, dietary fibre. Many of these substances are indispensable because they are not formed in the body but come only with food. The absence of at least one of them, for example, vitamin C, leads to illness and even death. Group B vitamins we receive mainly with bread from whole meal flour, and the source of vitamin A and other fat-soluble vitamins are dairy products, fish oil, and liver. Not each of us knows that we need to learn the culture of reasonable consumption, refrain from temptation, take another piece of a delicious product that gives extra calories, or introduces an imbalance. After all, any deviation from the laws of proper nutrition leads to a violation of health. The human body consumes energy not only during physical activity (during work, playing sports, etc.) but also in a state of relative rest (during sleep, lying down) when energy is used to maintain the physiological functions of the body - keeping constant body temperature. It was found that in a healthy middle-aged person with average body weight, 7 kilocalories per hour is consumed per kilogram of body weight. The first rule in any natural food system should be: - eating only with hunger; It is imperative to have free time for the assimilation of food. The idea that post- eating exercise promotes digestion is a blunder. Eating should consist of mixed foods that are sources of proteins, fats and carbohydrates, vitamins and minerals. Only in this case, it is possible to achieve a balanced ratio of nutrients and indispensable nutrition factors, to ensure not only a high level of digestion and absorption of nutrients but also their transportation to tissues and cells, their complete assimilation at the cell level. Synthetic nutrition ensures proper growth and formation of the body, contributes to maintaining health, high efficiency and prolonging life.

Peruse Progressively About How You Can Utilize Hypnotherapy to Treat

Welcome to hypnotherapy 101! If you've faltered your way here through a labyrinth of befuddling and opposing on the web sources, join the club. While trance and Hypnotherapy gloat establishes in old history and reams of tentatively checked outcomes, falsehood and folklore about the ideas flourish. As a prepared, affirmed, and rehearsing psychotherapist, you've learned how to search out top-notch, science-based solutions to your inquiries. Yet, straight answers about mesmerizing and Hypnotherapy can be rare.So how about we start at the earliest reference point.

What Is Spellbinding?

Mesmerizing is the demonstration of directing somebody into the unconscious state. Various specialists unexpectedly characterize the unconscious state, yet they quite often allude to:
A secret government of unwinding. Hyper focus and concentration.

Expanded Suggestibility

On the off chance that that sounds typical, this is because it is. A large portion of us goes all through the dazed state consistently. On the of a chance that you've at any point daydreamed on your everyday drive, fell into a dream while tuning in to music, or wound up drenched in the realm of a book or film, you've been in the unconscious state.(Find seven different ways you've been spellbound without acknowledging it.)The main contrast among entrancing and these regular daze states is that, in mesmerizing, somebody incites the unconscious state to accomplish something: mending, disclosure, or stress help, for instance.

What Isn't Trance?

Shouldn't something is said about where the trance inducer fools you into quacking like a duck or making their malicious offering? The possibility that subliminal specialists can assume control over their subjects' brains and control their activities is, obviously, an altogether media-driven fantasy. In the unconscious state, you control the entirety of your actions, you can hear everything around you, and you can't be compelled to accomplish something without wanting to. Affirmed trance specialist Cassie Salewske expresses, "In a hypnotherapy meeting, customers are cognizant; they are wakeful, taking an interest, and recalling. "Trance, she calls attention to, is known for outfitting "the intensity of proposal." However, it's not the first time our psyches are defenseless to the recommendation. Language and correspondence are immersed with the guidance," Salewske composes. Indeed, even members in stage subliminal therapy shows work heavily influenced by their personalities, as it's outlandish for somebody not to be aware while in a trance.

What Is Best Hypnotherapy?

To understand the contrast between spellbinding and hypnotherapy, consider trance an instrument and hypnotherapy to utilize an apparatus. In SAT terms, hypnotherapy is to sleep induction as craftsmanship treatment is to artistry. The meaning of hypnotherapy is evident from the word itself. Hypnotherapy is the act of entrancing for medicinal purposes. If you are an expert emotional health specialist or clinical specialist and you're utilizing entrancing to enable a customer to defeat a psychological or state of being, you're rehearsing hypnotherapy. The entrancing stupor state is a surprisingly adaptable apparatus for taking care of mental and physical medical issues. Here are only a couple of ways psychological health and clinical experts use hypnotherapy: Helping individuals quit smoking or lessen gorging by centering their psyches and recommending more beneficial conduct.

Getting to the psyche body connect to soothe constant and intense agony, including during medical procedure and labor. Hypnotherapy has likewise demonstrated powerful against onerous physical burdens like crabby inside disorder and dermatological conditions. I am jumping profound into the psyche brain to reveal and treat the underlying drivers of psychological health issues, for example, sadness, tension, PTSD, and fixation. We'll center the remainder of this article on that last use. The same number of trance specialists have found, the unconscious state is the way to opening the concealed profundities of our brains, recollections, and inspirations. (You would be shocked how regularly hypnotherapy is utilized in present-day medication and psychotherapy. Realize why specialists and advisors are going to hypnotherapy in our free whitepaper, "A definitive Manual for Clinical Hypnotherapy Methods.")

Accomplishes Hypnotherapy Work? What Does the Science State?

Since it gives moment access to the psyche mind, numerous specialists see hypnotherapy as more proficient than conventional treatment methods. "Hypnotherapy permits us to drop underneath the discerning piece of our psyche," clarifies trance specialist Stacie Shaft Bruce. Hypnotherapy gets to those passionate convictions that are going crazy. "We talked with 23 expert trance inducers as of late, and each revealed that hypnotherapy had changed their training and the lives of their customers. You can peruse their accounts in our free digital book. However, there is more than episodic proof that hypnotherapy works. The American Mental Affiliation closes, Even though spellbinding has been disputable, most clinicians currently concur it very well may be an incredible, viable restorative method for a broad scope of conditions, including agony, uneasiness, and mindset issue.

The English Mental Society charged a working gathering to review the proof and compose a proper report on hypnotherapy in 2001 and issues experienced in the act of medication, psychiatry, and psychotherapy. Front line cerebrum imaging innovation presently gives us a window into the physical signs of hypnotherapy. At the point when they examined the cerebrums of 57 people experiencing spellbinding, Stanford specialists announced that areas of the mind related to understanding and change indicated "modified movement and availability." (Hypnotherapy is a proof- based mental and physical health treatment method. Peruse the science with our free 140-page aggregation of mesmerizing and hypnotherapy references.)

What Emotional Health Issues Would Hypnotherapy Be Able to Help With?

A considerable lot of the hypnotherapists prepared by the Health Foundation have seen hypnotherapy as best against issues originating from curbed injury. Been frequenting them in a manner that appeared just as they were continually remembering that damaging second," Vitale says.

Hypnotherapist Wendy Pugh reveals to us hypnotherapy works incredibly well when youth injury has happened. Present working," she says. For instance, Pugh says, numerous individuals don't understand how profoundly their current tensions are established in occasions of the past.

By testing the past, covered feelings, and the bogus ends secured your customers' inner mind minds, you can utilize hypnotherapy to treat the absolute generally weakening and persistent emotional wellness challenges.

- PTSD

- Depression

- Migraines

- Performance tension

- Addictions

- Weight issues

- Anxiety and stress

- OCD

- Grief

- Cancer

- Childbirth

- Sleep

- Dementia

How Accomplishes Hypnotherapy Work with Different Modalities?

 It likewise encourages the utilization of stupor in progressively standard configurations." When hypnotherapy has opened up the entryway to your customers' subdued recollections and feelings — previous months or long periods of strenuous talk treatment — you can set yourself to the assignment of recuperating utilizing your time-tested strategies. Intellectual conduct treatment (CBT), specifically, is a viable supplement to hypnotherapy.

In our ongoing report, we investigated how the two modalities are regularly the most grounded working pair. We discussed ongoing logical investigations that have shown hypnotherapy is an advantageous aide to CBT for advancing weight loss and rewarding issues like bulimia nervosa and dissociative personality disorder.

Proves That Hypnosis Is Beneficial

Investigate my eyes. The expression brings to mind pictures of a psychotherapist swinging a pocket watch. Or, on the other hand, perhaps you picture Catherine Quicker in the film Get Out, tapping her teacup and sending a reluctant man into a condition of sleep-inducing limbo.

"There are numerous fantasies about hypnosis, for the most part originating from media introductions," like anecdotal movies and books, says Irving Kirsch, a speaker, and executive of the Program in Fake treatment Studies at Harvard Clinical School. Be that as it may, putting aside mainstream society buzzwords, Kirsch says hypnosis is a very much contemplated and real type of assistant treatment for conditions going from heftiness and torment after a medical procedure to uneasiness and stress. As far as weight loss, a portion of Kirsch's exploration has discovered that, contrasted with individuals experiencing intellectual conduct treatment (CBT)— one of the most proof sponsored non-tranquilize medicines for weight loss, gloom, and numerous different conditions—the individuals who experience psychological conduct treatment combined with hypnosis will, in general, lose more weight permanently. After four to six months, those suffering CBT+hypnosis dropped more than 20 pounds, while the individuals who simply did CBT lost about a large portion of that sum. The hypnosis bunch likewise kept up that weight loss during an 18-

month follow-up period, while the CBT-just gathering would, in general, recapture some weight.

Aside from supporting weight loss, there is "generous research proof" that hypnosis can successfully diminish physical torment, says Len Processing, a clinical psychologist and educator of brain research at the College of Hartford. One of Processing's audit articles found that hypnosis could help lessen children's post-careful agony or torment identified with other clinical systems. Another of his audit articles found that with regards to work and delivery-related suffering, hypnosis can at times altogether add to the advantages of standard clinical consideration—including epidurals and medications.

 David Spiegel, a hypnosis master and teacher of psychiatry and conduct sciences at Stanford College Institute of Medication. Found that 20% of individuals who got hypnosis figured out how to stop, contrasted with 14% of those accepting standard conduct guiding. The smoking suspension benefits were significantly progressively articulated among smokers with a history of grief—indicating an extra potential advantage of hypnosis.

Beneficial

Hypnosis can likewise be "beneficial" in rewarding pressure, uneasiness, and PTSD, Spiegel says. Research has discovered hypnosis can even change an individual's safe capacity in manners that counterbalance force and decrease weakness to viral contaminations.

Hypnosis involves, and how can it give these advantages? That's the place things get somewhat cloudy. Nearly everyone in the field concurs that the act of hypnosis includes two phases, which are typically alluded to as "acceptance" and "proposal."

This stage could last anyplace from a couple of moments to 10 minutes or more, and the objective of acceptance is to calm the psyche and concentrate on the therapist or instructor's voice and guidance. The "recommendation" stage includes talking the mesmerized individual through speculative occasions and situations expected to support that person address or balance unhelpful practices and feelings. Patients are welcome to encounter nonexistent incidents as though they were genuine, Processing says. The sort of proposals utilized relies upon the patient and his or her one of a kind difficulties.

Substantive Responses

Here and there, hypnosis can be contrasted with guided reflection or care; the thought is to put aside typical decisions and substantive responses and to enter a more profound condition of focus and responsiveness. Both Processing and Spiegel contrast hypnosis with losing oneself in a book or film—those occasions when the outside world blurs away, and an individual's psyche is caught in what she's perusing or viewing. Research has additionally alluded to hypnosis as the impermanent "decimation" of the inner self. Rather than permitting agony, nervousness, or other unhelpful states to manage everything, anesthesia causes individuals to apply more command over their considerations and discernments. How does hypnosis do this? Spiegel's exploration has indicated it can follow up on different cerebrum areas, including some connected to torment discernment and guideline. Hypnosis has likewise been found to calm pieces of the cerebrum associated with tangible Preparing and enthusiastic reaction. In any case, there's a great deal of discussion over how hypnosis functions, Processing says. "Initially, Freud estimated that hypnosis debilitates the boundary between the cognizant and subliminal," he says, including that this hypothesis has generally been deserted. While some property the intensity of hypnosis to the misleading impact, another theory is that "hypnosis makes individuals enter a changed condition of awareness, which makes them very receptive to entrancing

57

recommendations," he says. While talking about "adjusted conditions of awareness" sounds somewhat creepy, there's no loss of cognizance or amnesia. Not everyone benefits similarly from hypnosis. Processing says that regarding 20% of individuals show an "enormous" reaction to it, while a similar level doesn't react much by any stretch of the imagination. The staying half to 60% of individuals land someplace in the middle." Spiegel says. Be that as it may, even individuals who score low on proportions of sleep-inducing suggestibility can profit by it, Kirsch includes. He additionally means it's critical to see hypnosis as an enhancement to different types of treatment—something to be attempted uniquely related to CBT, psychotherapy, or different sorts of treatment.

Processing Emphasizes

Processing emphasizes this point. He thinks about specialists who are prepared distinctly in hypnosis to artisans who just expertise to utilize one device seeing an authorized clinician, instead of somebody who only practices hypnosis, is that the treatment is bound to be secured by protection.)

At last, don't anticipate that hypnosis should work after a solitary meeting. A few specialists state one shot can be viable. Be that as it may, Processing contends that "when all is said in done, a solitary treatment meeting including hypnosis is probably not going to be helpful."

It moreover energizes the usage of daze in logically standard designs." When hypnotherapy has opened up the gateway to your clients' quelled memories and emotions — earlier months or significant stretches of exhausting talk treatment — you can set yourself to the task of recovering using your tried and true procedures. Scholarly lead treatment (CBT), explicitly, is a feasible enhancement to hypnotherapy.

In our progressing report, we explored how the two modalities are routinely the most grounded working pair. We talked about progressing intelligent examinations that have demonstrated hypnotherapy is a favorable assistant to CBT for propelling weight decrease and compensating issues like bulimia nervosa and dissociative character issues.

Demonstrates That Spellbinding Is Gainful

Examine my eyes. The articulation infers photos of a psychotherapist swinging a pocket watch. Or, then again, maybe you picture Catherine Speedier in the film Get Out, tapping her teacup and sending a hesitant man into a state of rest actuating limbo.

"There are various dreams about spellbinding, generally starting from media presentations," like episodic films and books, says Irving Kirsch, a speaker, and official of the Program in Counterfeit treatment Studies at Harvard Clinical School. Nevertheless, setting aside standard society trendy expressions, Kirsch says entrancing is a particularly mulled over and genuine sort of right-hand treatment for conditions going from heaviness and torment after a clinical methodology to disquiet and stress. To the extent weight decrease, a part of Kirsch's investigation has found that, diverged from people encountering scholarly lead treatment (CBT)— one of the most confirmation supported non-sedate medications for weight decrease, despair, and various conditions—the people who experience direct mental treatment joined with a spellbinding will when all is said in done, lose more weight for all time. Following four to a half year, those enduring CBT+hypnosis dropped more than 20 pounds, while the people who just did CBT lost about a massive part of that entirety. The mesmerizing bundle similarly kept up that weight decrease during an 18-month follow-up period, while the CBT-simply assembling would recover some weight when all is said in done.

Weight Decrease

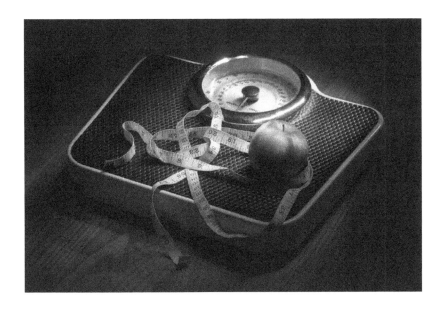

Besides supporting weight decrease, there is "liberal examination verification" that entrancing can effectively reduce physical torment, says Len Handling, a clinical analyst and instructor of cerebrum research at the School of Hartford. One of Preparing's review articles found that entrancing could help diminish youngsters' post-cautious anguish or torment related to other clinical frameworks. Another of his review articles found that concerning work and conveyance connected misery, trance can now and again through and through add to the benefits of standard clinical thought—including epidurals and prescriptions.

David Spiegel, an entrancing expert, and instructor of psychiatry and direct sciences at Stanford School Organization of Prescription. Discovered that 20%

of people who got trance made sense of how to stop, appeared differently about 14% of those tolerating standard lead directing. The smoking suspension benefits were altogether dynamically enunciated among smokers with a background marked by sadness—showing an additional likely favorable position of mesmerizing. Spellbinding can, in like manner, be "advantageous" in compensating weight, disquiet, and PTSD, Spiegel says. The examination has found trance can even change a person's protected limit inhabits that balance power and abatement shortcoming to viral pollutions. Spellbinding include, and how might it give these points of interest? That is the spot things get to some degree cloudy. Nearly everybody in the field agrees that the demonstration of trance incorporates two stages, which are commonly mentioned as "acknowledgment" and "proposition."

Incorporates

This stage could last wherever from two or three minutes to 10 minutes or more, and the target of acknowledgment is to quiet the mind and focus on the specialist or educator's voice and direction. The "suggestion" stage incorporates talking the entranced individual through theoretical events and circumstances expected to help that individual location or parity unhelpful practices and sentiments. Patients are free to experience nonexistent occurrences just as they were authentic, Preparing says. The kind of proposition used depends upon the patient and their stand-out troubles.

To a great extent, entrancing can stand out from guided reflection or care; the idea is to set aside usual choices and meaningful reactions and enter an increasingly significant state of center and responsiveness. Both Preparing and Spiegel balance spellbinding with losing oneself in a book or film—those events when the outside world foggy spots away, and a person's mind is trapped in what she's examining or survey. The examination has furthermore insinuated mesmerizing as the temporary "annihilation" of the internal identity. As opposed to allowing desolation, apprehension, or other unhelpful states to oversee everything, sedation makes people apply for more orders over their contemplations and observations. How does trance do this? Spiegel's investigation has demonstrated it can catch up on various cerebrum zones, including some associated with torment insight and rule. Mesmerizing has moreover been found to quiet bits of the cerebrum related with unmistakable getting ready and energetic response.

Handling Stresses

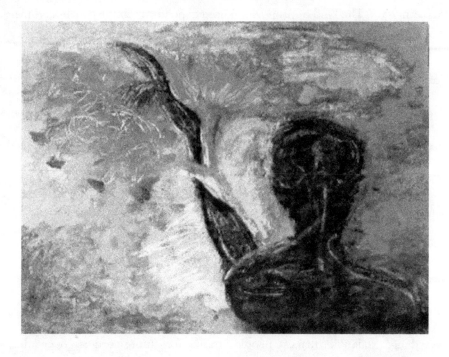

Regardless, there's a lot of conversation over how spellbinding capacities, Handling says. "At first, Freud evaluated that mesmerizing incapacitates the limit between the discerning and subconscious," he says, including that this speculation has commonly been abandoned. While some property the force of mesmerizing to the deceptive effect, another hypothesis is that "spellbinding causes people to enter a changed state of mindfulness, which makes them open to enchanting proposals," he says. While discussing "balanced states of mindfulness" sounds to some degree unpleasant, there's no loss of awareness or amnesia. Not every person benefits comparatively from spellbinding. Preparing says that concerning

20% of people show a "gigantic" response to it, while a similar level doesn't respond much in any way, shape, or form. The remaining half to 60% of people lands somewhere in the center." Spiegel says. In any case, even people who score low on extents of rest instigating suggestibility can benefit by it, Kirsch incorporates. He furthermore implies it's essential to consider spellbinding to be an upgrade to various kinds of treatment—something to be endeavored remarkably identified with CBT, psychotherapy, or different sorts of treatment.

Handling stresses this point. He considers masters who are arranged unmistakably in entrancing to artisans who only mastery to use one gadget seeing an approved clinician, rather than someone who just practices trance, is that the treatment will undoubtedly be made sure about by insurance.) Finally, don't foresee that mesmerizing should work after a single gathering. A couple of expert's states one shot can be practical. In any case, preparing battles that "when everything is said in done, a singular treatment meeting including spellbinding is most likely not going to be useful."

Adjustment: August 31

The first form of this story misquoted the discoveries of two of Processing's audit articles. Hypnosis was found to fundamentally add to the advantages of standard clinical consideration, not outflank it. Hypnosis was additionally found to diminish children's post-careful torment, not to dispose of it. It likewise misrepresented Processing's perspective on the "recommendation" period of hypnosis. Recommendations are custom-fitted greeting to encounter nonexistent occasions as though they were genuine. They are not subject to the individual, and they dislike asking an analyst what they will say during psychotherapy.

The Progressively Open to Conversation and Proposal

- Phobias, fears, and tension

- Sleep issue

- Depression

- Stress

- Post-injury tension

- Grief and misfortune

Hypnosis likewise may be utilized to help with torment control and to beat propensities, for example, smoking or gorging. Severe or who need emergency the executives.

What Are the Downsides of Hypnosis?

Hypnosis probably won't be suitable for an individual who has insane indications, for example, mind flights used for torment control only after a specialist has assessed the individual for any physical issue that may require clinical or careful treatment. Hypnosis additionally might be a less powerful type of therapy than other increasingly customary medicines, for example, prescription, for mental disarranges. A few advisors use hypnosis to recuperate conceivably quelled recollections they accept are connected to the individual's psychological issue. In any case, the quality and unwavering quality of data reviewed by the patient under hypnosis aren't generally stable. Thus, hypnosis is not, at this point, considered a typical or standard piece of most types of psychotherapy. Likewise, the utilization of hypnosis for specific psychological issues wherein patients might be profoundly helpless to the recommendation, for example, dissociative scatters, remains particularly disputable.

Is Hypnosis Perilous?

Hypnosis is certainly not a dangerous method. It wouldn't fret control or programming. The most serious hazard, as discussed above, is that bogus recollections can conceivably be made and progressively settled, and conventional mental medicines.

Who Performs Hypnosis?

Hypnosis is performed by an authorized or affirmed emotional health proficient, who is exceptionally prepared in this method.

Human givens advisors, with well-meaning goals, are no uncertainty acclimated with survey hypnosis, anyway, we may term it, as a power for good. Utilizing this system can, for sure, lead to incredible therapeutic continuously used sensibly.

Sadly, something puzzling frequently appends itself to discuss hypnosis; even though hypnosis has been thought about for quite a long time and has been the subject of logical research for more than 200 years, there is yet across the board misjudging about what it is. A glance on the web raises a whole scope of thoughts, extensively dozing confused condition, "relapse in the administration of the sense of self," or a state of centered consideration) and 'non-state' speculations (it's merely play-acting).

Sorting Out Thought

We need a more significant sorting out thought, and the human givens give one: hypnosis isn't a condition of awareness by any means; it is any counterfeit methods for getting to the REM state. In this way, hypnosis is a procedure, separate from the daze express that it instigates, and its belongings are not, at this point, strange because this can represent all wonders related to it.

It is undeniable that hypnosis is a fake procedure, as opposed to a state, when we consider that we, as a rule, go into a daze Be that as it may, Also, in that lies the peril.

Any individual who can concentrate has a decent creative mind or can turn out to be genuinely excited will, at various focuses in time, enter stupor. We are in a self-incited stupor at whatever point we are profoundly sincerely stirred in what is generally thought of as a negative way: outrage, fierceness, scorn, dread, tension, stressing, sorrow, begrudge, avarice, narrow- mindedness. Every single such feeling cuts us off from our reasoning cerebrums and gives the music, moved by verse, craftsmanship, or show, to begin to look all starry eyed at or make energetic.

Utilizing Abilities

As a result, on programmed. For example, getting consumed in inventive exercises, cooking, cultivating, composting, making craftsmanship, music, verse or ceramics, singing, and moving, put us in a daze, as can peruse and examine. Exercises like singing and walking are exceptionally dazed initiating, additionally thoroughly retaining. We can even enter an unconscious state known as 'stream' when we realize how to accomplish something truly well. In doing that action, our feeling of having a different self-briefly vanishes, and we quickly become one with what we are doing. This kind of joyful daze, when we enter it, appears to work self-rulingly inside us: we become the experience that we are making. This exceptional ability to go into a stream, which a few analysts call a 'top understanding' and others depict as 'being in the zone,' contributes a lot to the feeling of life being significant.

Daze can likewise be instigated, purposefully or something else, by drugs, stun, slow ceremonies, sleep-inducing language, startling touch, petition, sexual action, reflection, gazing, being approached to review specific recollections, voracity, changing breathing examples to be sure, any boost that stimulates compelling feeling and, incomprehensibly, any type of profound unwinding that brings down passionate excitement. The three most fundamental structures, creatures experience as well, are dreaming, getting profoundly emotional, and learning and none require entrancing acceptance.

Condition of Consideration

How an engaged state of attention is created can have an immediate bearing on the quality, profundity, and length of a daze. For instance, one purpose behind structure wonderfully excellent houses of prayer, mosques, sanctuaries, and castles stupor condition of stunningness, which made them profoundly suggestible and all the more tolerating of whatever lessons or guidelines were granted to them in those situations. Also, when individuals wear covers, they go into stupor act in manners by which they would not typically carry on, concentrating consideration on this feeling of change. The most profound daze of all, Human given's information about the whole idea of trance and hypnosis gets from the desire satisfaction hypothesis of Joe Griffin's dreams.1 For, the most profound stupor of everything is dreaming. It is the essential type of daze that creates in the belly when the embryo's first beginnings are the initiation of a particular mind circuit, known as ponto- geniculate-occipital (PGO) waves.) It was rest investigate pioneer Michel Jouvet, presently an emeritus teacher of trial medication at the College of Lyon, who had the exceptional understanding that it is during REM rest that impulses are modified trustworthiness of our inspirations. For dreams are allegorical interpretations of sincerely stirring desires not followed upon in the past waking time frame. Dreams deactivate the passionate excitement, liberating the mind to react anew to each new day in this manner, keeping up the respectability of our senses.

<u>REM</u>

Daze as the REM state due to the away from likenesses with the territory of REM rest. When acting by entrancing, a profound stupor mirrors various pieces of REM rest, for instance, invulnerability to unmistakable outside information, less affectability to torment, muscle loss of movement, etc. Likewise, portions of how the REM state limits when we long for equivalent methodologies used for starting surprise. Many daze inducers may utilize melodic improvement to help make daze (for instance, making dull hand advancements or getting people to look at turning optical mind flights), which associations back to the rough fish cerebrum that we progressed from. (Fish blow up to musicality because of their likely need to move, steer, and level cutting edges.) Focusing thought mirrors ingestion in a dream. Another comparability is toward consideration: causing a boisterous disturbance or lopsided advancement that can put a person into a trance, like that in a brief moment, get their thought and incorporates electrical brain activity known as the immediate response identical PGO waves as found in REM rest. Exactly when we initially start to dream, the course response fires angrily. The craving fulfillment theory of dreams explains this is the segment for making the cerebrum mindful of the proximity of unexpressed enthusiastic sentiments of energy that need discharging in a dream.

There are yet more resemblances. The significant loosening up, which psychotherapists use as enrollment into a daze, matches what happens as we fall asleep. Additionally, when clients are free, the guided imagery we use to engage them to comprehend their difficulties from with a superior perspective and destruction them matches dream material developing the qualification being that, in a misleadingly impelled trance, the pro is controlling the methodology, while unacted-out energetic sentiments of energy from the previous day give the 'dream content imagery' in our rest. As we presumably know, the similarity is strange in treatment when given to a person in a surprise; and dreams are portrayals. Express surprise experiences may incorporate perceptions clients may report 'feeling' everywhere throughout the shine illusory. Exploration has shown that comparative brain pathways are dynamic in the two conditions. Moreover, wonders that can be actuated in surprise are similarly quickly experienced in dreaming, for instance, amnesia (for the dream), sedation and nonappearance of agony, body dreams, catalepsy, partition, and time-turning.

Additionally, as enchanting isn't the shock, in any case, so the REM state isn't the dream. It is, basically, the theater where the sentiment occurs. As Joe Griffin showed up, the dream content is separated from the REM theater, our inward 'reality generator,' and is continued, or made certified, inside it.

REM State

The REM state, by then, is dynamic in a full scope of surprise. It isn't just a 'free' or 'dormant' state. It is dynamic. It is locked in with programming fundamental and taught data full scope of learning, scholastics, or something different (checking treatment, trim, and teaching) and when we stray in dreamland and deal with issues. Right when we are being harmed, the REM state is the medium through which the horrendous mishap is gotten by the cerebrum and transforms into an adjusted bit of the perseverance positions. So, the REM state is necessary to see, primarily if we are related to passing on treatment. Mirrors different bits of REM rest, for example, immunity to outside unquestionable data, less affectability to torment, muscle loss of development, and so forth. In like manner, parts of how the REM state limits when we long for proportionate strategies utilized for beginning amazement. Many shock inducers may use melodic improvement to help make a surprise (for example, making dull hand headways or getting individuals to take a gander at turning optical psyche flights), which relates to the harsh fish cerebrum that we advanced from. (Fish explode to musicality based on their anticipated need to move, steer, and level forefronts.) Centering thought mirrors ingestion in a fantasy. Another similarity is toward thinking: causing an uproarious unsettling influence or disproportionate progression that can place an individual into a daze. Like that in a brief second,

74

get their idea and join the electrical mind movement known as the quick reaction indistinguishable PGO waves as found in REM rest. Precisely when we at first begin to dream, the course reaction fires irately. The hankering satisfaction hypothesis of dreams clarifies this is the section for making the cerebrum aware of the vicinity of unexpressed energetic assessments of vitality that need releasing in a dream.

There are yet more likenesses. The huge extricating up, which psychotherapists use as an enlistment into a shock, match what occurs as we nod off. Furthermore, when customers are free, the guided symbolism we use to connect with them to appreciate their troubles from with a predominant viewpoint and annihilation them matches dream material creating the capability being that, in a misleadingly actuated stupor, the expert is controlling the technique, while unacted-out enthusiastic conclusions of vitality from the earlier day give the 'fantasy content symbolism' in our rest. As we probably know, the similitude is weird in treatment when given to an individual in astonishment; and dreams are depictions. Express astonishment encounters may consolidate observations customers may report 'feeling' wherever all through the sparkle deceptive. The investigation has indicated that relative mind pathways are dynamic in the two conditions. Also, ponders that can be activated in shock are likewise They are immediately experienced in dreaming, for example, amnesia (for the fantasy), sedation and nonappearance of distress, body dreams, catalepsy, parcel, and time-turning.

Rem State Isn't the Fantasy

As charming isn't the stun, regardless, the REM state isn't the fantasy. It is, essentially, the theater where the slant internal 'reality generator,' and is proceeded or made ensured, inside it.

The REM state, by at that point, is dynamic in a full extent of shock. It isn't only a 'free' or 'lethargic' state. It is dynamic. It is secured with programming key and showed information a full extent of learning, scholastics, or something else (checking treatment, trim, and educating) and when we stray in fantasy land and manage issues. Right when we are being hurt, the REM state is the medium through which the repulsive accident is gotten by the cerebrum and changes into a balanced piece of the tirelessness positions. So, the REM state is fundamental to see, particularly if we are connected with passing on treatment.

The Advancement of Befuddling Misleading Statements

A misleading statement is similarly as dangerous as a falsehood, regardless of whether offering the right rambled about trance, and professionals should be mindful so as not to declare them. They incorporate the accompanying.

¨ "Hypnosis is a characteristic condition of unwinding and fixation, with uplifted mindfulness incited by the proposal."

¨ It isn't. As I have depicted, it is a counterfeit method for getting to the REM state, which should even be possible savagely by catching consideration with an unexpected noisy commotion or frightening development.

¨ "Hypnosis is sheltered with no terrible reactions."

¨ It is a long way from safe. It is an incredibly fantastic procedure, and anything ground-breaking can be utilized to do hurt just as high. A few people feel doubtful or uncomfortable, considerably after a loosening up meeting. They may feel mentally alarmed about being 'wild,' especially if they didn't care for the recommendations that were made to them. The writing is loaded with terrible or even hazardous impacts that have been experienced after the trance. They incorporate extreme weariness; reserved carrying on; nervousness; alarm assaults; consideration shortfall; body/mental self-view contortions; appreciation/fixation misfortune; disarray; hindered adapting abilities; fanciful reasoning; sadness; depersonalization; wooziness; dreadfulness; migraine; a sleeping disorder; fractiousness; impeded or mutilated memory; queasiness and regurgitating; Sometimes, that is the situation when somebody is in a slight daze, however, frequently specialist said. This shouldn't imply that they didn't enroll in it. Yet, they can't intentionally review it.

¨ "Hypnosis has nothing to do with rest it is only an amazingly loosened upstate."

¨ Clearly, this isn't right since trance is legitimately

Historical Backdrop

We know basically by digging into the historical backdrop of entrancing of numerous instances of undesirable impact. There are multiple current episodes, some of which are recorded on CCTV cameras, for example, clerks being entranced and giving over the cash in their tills since they were placed into a stupor state, or individuals being stunned into a daze an exquisite, caring tone, on a YouTube video. The oblivious isn't insightful by any stretch of the imagination. It is primarily impacted by how we are raised, our background and the way of life we live in, etc.: our molding. Most definitely, the GIGO rule applies: trash in, trash out. A significant part of the therapeutic work done in a daze is worried about abrogating programmed oblivious reactions, changing unfortunate

78

examples, and opening up restricted discernments.

- Experts of the entrancing need to recognize and secure against.

- Taking somebody's feeling of volition endlessly.

- We realize that feeling a feeling of authority over our own lives is a natural human need. It isn't the therapists' place to make suspicions about what a customer need. In this manner, it is exceptionally significant that any progressions a customer is guided to make, having been prompted into a stupor state, are as per objectives built up already and comprehended by both customer and specialist. It ought to likewise be our plan to give our customers the devices to adapt without us, as fast as could be expected under the circumstances. In this way, it is significant for specialists to ace successful no longer need treatment.

- Muddied expectation

Specialist Conveying

The expectation of the specialist conveying the mediation is hugely significant as far as results. Surely, if there is an earnest expectation to enable an individual, even an advisor who isn't, in fact, gigantically capable can get a decent outcome. In any case, uncommon are the individuals who can set their personalities aside and that implies uncommon among advisors as well. Inner self can introduce a specific entanglement for some who use hypnotherapy, as they have found that it is difficult to place individuals into a daze, though, to the vast majority, it appears to be a baffling tremendous aptitude and explicit dirty tricks, including arm levitation, so their self-images puff up, which is enormously harming trance is to forestall confusion concerning both advisor and customer.) Luckily, one of our natural assets, which is an integral self.' At a logical level, this mindfulness happens when we unwind. The neocortex can work without inordinate enthusiastic impedance. It empowers us to take a gander at reality all the more equitably and perceive on the off chance that we are excessively diverted with ourselves.

- Creating bogus (fanciful) recollections

- Inducing mind flights

- Which can lead powerless individuals into crazy breakdowns. This is the stock in exchange for the stage subliminal specialist. It's perilous because an individual in an insane state

- Includes all cliques and ideological groups polish the REM state, and, somehow, entrancing. For instance, the utilization by government officials of powerful sleep-inducing words like 'constructive change,' 'qualities' or 'standards,' power individuals into an inside daze to scan for what they comprehend as the importance of these words through the Furthermore, no individual needs a negative change. So, when a government official uses words like change or dynamic, it is a con stunt.)

Mesmerizing Is Innocuous

Anyone who thinks mesmerizing is innocuous may do well to recollect that Hitler examined it in the wake of being restored by a subliminal specialist of the crazy visual deficiency that he endured toward the finish of the Principal Universal proposal given in daze by a therapist who disclosed to him that he was exceptional and that he had extraordinary individual forces and that, with these incredible forces, he could fix himself of the visual impairment. This went about as a trancelike post recommendation, and Hitler proceeded to actuate responsive daze states in large groups at rallies, assaulting them with sincerely stirring nominalizations. He even received a stylized type of arm levitation as the Nazi salute.

Obviously, in treatment, vague language is utilized with benevolent goals, to send customers on their interior quest to discover implications for 'internal assets,' 'inventiveness' and 'qualities' and so forth, very well may be shockingly simple to be enticed into a stupor, in any event, when you think you know better.

- Unwanted clairvoyance

- Therapists will, in general, go into a profoundly engaged state when they are sincerely attempting to support someone, and, at such minutes, the disarray of sense of self-limits can happen, hurting both advisors enormous bang.2

Numerous specialists experience clairvoyance with their customers. For example, if an advisor, for reasons unknown, is feeling less than impressive and wishes that they had fewer customers that day, customers will frequently begin to ring up and delay arrangements. It is bewildering and occurs extremely regularly to be down to risk. (A related, healthy experience is that of abruptly worthy to assault, torment, and murder individuals surely, exceptionally suggestible. All perilous mass developments include entrancing and the programming of individuals, when they are genuinely stimulated.

• This peril has, for some time, been known. As the prestigious Indian Hindu priest Master Vivekananda stated, "Think about the brain like a group of wild ponies, and as opposed customary meetings of mesmerizing from someone else, going into this compliant state, rather than picking up force and better control, the brain can turn into an undefined frail mass, inevitably prompting the psychological haven." A rendition of this is the thing that may occur if specialists over and over an attempt to support a mentally harmed individual by disclosing to them that they are capable of Thoughtless utilization of spellbinding can meddle with individuals' mental and profound turn of events. It isn't exaggerated to call that mystic homicide.

Utilizing the REM state in treatment

We can observe how trance fits with the APET™ model of enacting specialist, design coordinating, feeling, and thought. The enacting specialist in whatever implies the advisors decides for initiating the REM state in the customer (we suggest delicate ways, not brutal ways, similar to stun). The customer's cerebrum design matches the pleasant thoughts proposed by the advisor and gives them individual significance. Each example coordinates flames an enthusiastic reaction (a desire), anyway unobtrusive.

The Phases of Powerful Hypnotherapy

These Are:

- Induction: falsely

- That person for learning

- Educate: manage the customer's

- Consideration and include new information that gives their life a more extravagant setting. All learning occurs in a daze. At whatever point we perceive something natural on the planet, it is consistently because of the earth, and an inside put away the case, which we ordinarily call a memory. Our minds are continually design coordinating to the outside world, and we possibly become mindful of that if something other than what's expected from the standard happens the direction reaction fires and our consideration is attracted to it. All learning, by its inclination, includes oddity, and we need to center, anyway quickly, on what's happening and consumed is significant, we have to introspect about this unique example coordinate and modify our model of reality to it. In this way, all learning is post-sleep inducing.

- Heal help realize mental mending by directing an individual to get to positive life assets and tackle the psychological procedures expected to practice solid new practices; and physical recuperating, by aiding or persuading the body to mend itself.

- Ensure volition: give full oversight back to the customer.

- First, make no mischief.

- The uprightness of the individual doing the treatment

- The specialist's genuineness and knowledge (enthusiastic and something else)

- Their level of ability and how well they use language aptitudes; particularly similitude

- The advisor's degree of mental information and self-information

- Their comprehension of intrinsic enthusiastic needs about what a patient indeed requires

- The advisor's capacity to set their sense of self aside

- Nature

Positive Affirmations for Weight Loss to Reach Your Fitness Goals

Even though this was a little report, comparative investigations all show that fat patients improve at diminishing worry with care works out. Their outcomes offer an interesting gander at how reflection rehearses for pressure decrease may help lessen the hormone cortisol levels, with a related drop in stomach fat without customary consuming fewer calories. Past creature examines have discovered a connection between stress eating and where fat is kept. Food inclinations (even in rodents) move under worry to devouring progressively fat, and sugar, with vitality, put away as fat moving to the body's midriff. The scientists state their investigation recommends that careful preparation in people may assist them with adapting better to pressure and other antagonistic feelings, which could lead to more beneficial dissemination of muscle versus fat from eating better and loosening up additional.

Hypnosis for Naturally Weight Loss

What Is Hypnosis for Weight Loss and Accomplishes

It Work?

Regarding getting in shape, you think about the standard go-to experts: specialists, nutritionists, dietitians, fitness coaches, and even psychological health the one you haven't precisely thought of yet: a subliminal specialist. It turns out utilizing hypnosis is another street individual are wandering down for the sake of weight loss. Furthermore, commonly, it's gone after the various final desperate attempts (I see you, juice purifies, and prevailing fashion eats less) are attempted and fizzled, says Greg Gurniak, a confirmed clinical and clinical trance specialist rehearsing in Ontario.

Hypnosis," says Kimberly Friedmutter, trance inducer and creator of Subconscious Force: Utilize Your Inward Psyche to Make the Existence You've Generally Needed.

You're likewise not oblivious when you experience hypnosis—it's increasingly similar to a secret government of unwinding, Friedmutter clarifies the day before you're which is why hypnosis for weight loss might be powerful. Recollections, propensities, fears, food affiliations, negative self-talk, and confidence grow," says

86

Capri Cruz, Ph.D., psychotherapist, and trance specialist and creator of Augment Your Super Powers.

In Any Case, Does Hypnosis for Weight Loss Work?

There isn't a massive amount of later, randomized research accessible regarding the matter; however, what is out there proposes that the strategy could be conceivable. Early examinations from the 90s found that individuals who utilized hypnosis lost more than twice as much weight as those who consumed fewer calories without psychological treatment. Furthermore, a little 2017 investigation worked with eight overweight, maintaining a strategic distance from the medical procedure because of the treatment benefits. None of this is convincing.

Cruz says. Be that as it may, with the ever-expanding cost of physician recommended drugs, excellent arrangements of conceivable symptoms, and the push for increasingly characteristic other options, Cruz is positive hypnosis credible weight loss approach.

Who Should Attempt Hypnosis for Weight Loss?

The perfect up-and-comer is, indeed, destructive tendencies—like a subliminal issue. Your inner mind is the place your feelings, propensities, and addictions are found, Friedmutter says. Indeed, an investigation from 1970 discovered hypnosis to have a 93 percent achievement rate, with fewer sessions required than both psychotherapy and conduct treatment Gurniak says hypnosis can likewise be utilized as a commendation to other weight loss programs structured by experts to treat different health conditions, be it diabetes, stoutness, joint pain, or cardiovascular sickness. Sessions can differ long and technique relying upon the professional. Dr. Cruz, for instance, says her sessions regularly last somewhere in the range of 45 and an hour, though Friedmutter sees weight loss patients for three to four hours. In any case, as a rule, you can hope to set down, unwind with your eyes shut, and let the trance inducer control you through specific procedures and proposals that can assist you with arriving at your goals."The thought is to prepare the psyche to push toward what is sound and away based on what is undesirable," Friedmutter says.

Hypnosis Weight Loss Guided Sessions

Regarding getting in shape, you think about the typical go-to experts: specialists, nutritionists, dietitians, fitness coaches, and even psychological health, the one you haven't precisely thought of yet: a trance specialist. It turns out utilizing hypnosis is another street individual are wandering down for the sake of weight loss. Also, usually, it's gone after the various final desperate attempts (I see you, juice purifies, and trend counts calories) are attempted and fizzled, says Greg Gurniak, a guaranteed clinical and clinical trance inducer rehearsing in Ontario.

another person is controlling your brain and causing you to do entertaining things while you're oblivious. "Psyche control and losing control—otherwise known as accomplishing something without wanting to—are the greatest confusions about hypnosis," says Kimberly Friedmutter, trance specialist and creator of Subconscious Force: Utilize Your Internal Brain to Make the Existence You've Generally Needed. You're likewise not oblivious when you experience hypnosis—it's progressively similar to an underground government of unwinding, Friedmutter clarifies.

Being in that state makes you increasingly powerless to change, and that is the reason hypnosis for weight loss might be successful their recollections, propensities, fears, food affiliations, negative self-talk, and confidence sprout," says Capri Cruz, Ph.D., psychotherapist, and trance inducer and creator of Augment Your Super Powers.

In Any Case, Does Hypnosis for Weight Loss Work?

There aren't a ton of examinations from the 90s found that individuals who utilized hypnosis counted calories without intellectual treatment. A recent report worked with 60 hefty ladies and found that the individuals who rehearsed hypnobehavioral treatment shed pounds and improved their eating propensities and self-perception. And a little 2017 investigation worked with eight hefty grown-ups and three youngsters. Each of them effectively sheds pounds, with one, in any event, avoiding medical procedure because of the treatment benefits. None of this is convincing. Cruz says. In any case, with the ever-expanding cost of professionally prescribed medications, excellent arrangements of conceivable reactions, and the push for progressively regular other options, Cruz is cheerful hypnosis.

Who Should Attempt Hypnosis for Weight Loss?

The perfect candidate is a destructive tendency like eating the whole pack of potato chips instead of stopping when you're full—is an indication of a subliminal issue, he says. Your inner mind is the place your feelings, propensities, and addictions are found, Friedmutter says. And because hypnotherapy addresses the emotional mind—rather than merely the aware— it might be progressively viable. An investigation examination from 1970 discovered hypnosis to have a 93 percent achievement rate, with fewer meetings required than both psychotherapy and conduct treatment. **Gurniak says** hypnosis heftiness, joint inflammation, or cardiovascular sickness.

What Would I Be Able to Expect During A Treatment?

Meetings can fluctuate long, and strategy is relying upon the expert. Dr. Cruz, for instance, says her sessions usually. Yet, as a rule, you can hope to set down, unwind with your eyes shut, and let the trance inducer manage you through specific procedures and recommendations that can assist you with arriving at your objectives. food, we can figure out how to respect them. "And no, you won't cackle like a chicken or admitting any profound, dim insider facts. Instead, you'll experience a profound unwinding, while as yet monitoring what's being stated, Gurniak includes. We fill in as a group to accomplish the individual's objective. "The quantity of meetings required is reliant on your reaction to hypnosis. And on the other hand, it may not be viable for everybody. With the correct and strictly observed regimen, a bright and essential rhythm of the functioning of the body is developed, which creates optimal conditions for work and rest and thereby contributes to better health, better working capacity and higher labour productivity. The next link in a healthy lifestyle is the eradication of bad habits (smoking, alcohol, drugs). These health violators are the cause of many diseases, drastically reduce life expectancy, reduce efficiency, adversely affect the health of the younger generation and the health of future children.

The next component of a healthy lifestyle is a balanced diet. When it comes to it, you should remember two fundamental laws, the violation of which is dangerous to health. The first law is the equilibrium of the energy received and consumed. If the body gets more energy than it expends, that is, if we receive more food than is necessary for the healthy development of a person, work and well-being, we become fuller. The second law is "compliance of the chemical composition of the diet with the physiological needs of the body in nutrients". Nutrition should be varied and meet the needs for proteins, fats, carbohydrates, vitamins, minerals, dietary fibre. Many of these substances are indispensable because they are not formed in the body but come only with food. The absence of at least one of them, for example, vitamin C, leads to illness and even death. Group B vitamins we receive mainly with bread from wholemeal flour, and the source of vitamin A and other fat-soluble vitamins are dairy products, fish oil, and liver. It was found that in a healthy middle- aged person with average body weight, 7 kilocalories per hour is consumed per kilogram of body weight. The first rule in any natural food system should be: eating only with hunger; refusal to eat with pain, mental and physical malaise, with fever and elevated body temperature; refusal to eat immediately before bedtime, as well as before and after serious work, physical or mental. It is imperative to have free time for the assimilation of food. The idea that post-eating exercise promotes digestion is a blunder. Eating should consist of mixed foods that are sources of proteins, fats and carbohydrates, vitamins and minerals.

Hypnosis to Avoid Binge and Emotional Eating

Let's face it; the more significant part of us have utilized food to feel much improved. Regardless of whether it's deep plunging into Ben and Jerry's after you find his mystery sexts, or heading home with a double outside layer following a terrible day at the workplace, emotional eating happens to potentially anyone. It's a steady, day by day battle that keeps them from ever accomplishing a stable weight or effectively keeping off weight they do figure out how to lose. Emotionally activated eating implies that we use food to direct our feelings and attempting to stop it can feel unthinkable. I recall one well-known nutritionist letting me know: 'On the off chance that somebody is happy to focus on my program, I can assist anybody with getting thinner and get the body they had always wanted that is, except if they are an emotional eater. That is outlandish.'

As somebody who has utilized food to handle worry for a mind-blowing majority this was debilitating. I understand that getting more fit is feasible, having endeavored all way of diets from Keto and Paleo to Weight Watchers and Juice Rinse. Sour, I always act like I am going to discover the solutions to my issues at the bottom of a sack of Cool Farm Doritos. I recall my sister messaging me once after I'd had an especially untidy separation, saying: 'Recollect, Señor Dominos isn't your companion.'

Subliminal specialist and Holistic mentor Malminder Gill Subliminal specialist and holistic mentor Malminder Gill

<u>Food Longings</u>

Finding that UK subliminal specialist Malminder Gill, who has rewarded probably the most renowned faces on the planet, has a forte in helping beat emotional eating was entertaining. I went in questionable. I'd been mesmerized previously once to manage food longings and once for richness and the impacts endured all of around five minutes. This time was extraordinary.

Entering her Harley Road center, Gill comforts me right away. She oozes warmth. She begins by asking me a lot of inquiries about my youth, my connections, what is worrying me right now and what satisfies me. Her way is encouraging I have an inclination that I'm conversing with a companion. At that point, she begins to pose inquiries that revolved around my eating propensities. It feels like a doctor delicately looking around a touchy region attempting to make sense of what harms.

A lot of my customers battle with it. We will generally consider emotional eating as happening just when we're tragic or pushed. However, I have customers who eat emotionally when they're incredibly cheerful or even furious. She gets some information about my morning schedule saying it's the most significant second to make the change as it sets you up for the afternoon.

When she discovers I put artificial sugar in my espresso and incidentally, I have a dependence on diet Coke it resembles the penny drops. 'Ok. ' she says. 'You have to stop the fake. Did you realize that they give fake sugars to pigs to get them to eat more before they are butchered? It truly pushes them (and you) to eat more. It's just about the most noticeably awful thing you can do.'

Even though we're merely having a discussion I was not spellbound at all yet she refers to the big thing a couple of more occasions. I wind up in the coming days considering 'fat all pigs' events I see my cherished Pepsi Max on the grocery store rack. I don't get it.

<u>My Home Work</u>

My home work for the week is to kick back and see when I feel a food hankering. To feel it start, and to intellectually remain again and state to myself, 'goodness truly, this is a hankering happening at present,' to time it, believe it gets more grounded and feels its ebb. What's more, through the span of the following not many weeks, she figures out how to accomplish something nobody ever has in

15 years: Get me to quit drinking a day by day diet Coke and to quit improving my espresso. Our next meeting starts with entrancing, where she begins to handle the feelings.

Before we begin, she advises me that there is nothing but bad or terrible nourishments. 'I am dealing with raising your degree of goal when you eat. Eating isn't a response or an instrument to calm you yet an informed decision. I don't have confidence in eats less because they are brief arrangements. We have to make sense of your relationship to food, which drives you to utilize it for solace and find different approaches to complete it. That is, it.'

She calls her procedure 'Careful Eating' since she says it's not tied in with following a program precisely there are no nourishments beyond reach here it's about reprogramming your brain, so you eat from a position of expectation, not in response to something different. Gill says: 'I comprehend why individuals need to get more fit rapidly and take extreme apportions cutting whole nutrition types, disregarding carbs or rehearsing serious fasting. Be that as it may, I state, quit abstaining from excessive food intake altogether. Figure out how to quit eating due to feelings and get reacquainted with appetite and completion prompts.' As I lay with my eyes shut on a table in her faintly lit office, she starts in an alleviating, calm voice she discusses my propensities, feelings, and aim. I feel without a care in the world during the meeting. Gill has made a 'content' that is close to home to me and incorporates a great deal of the things I'd advised her. I am mindful of her voice when she discusses relinquishing the things that are keeping me away from the sound way of life, I need to live I am not snoozing precisely, yet I am incredible, loose. It feels like I've quite recently had an average portion of co codamol.

Top Tips to Beat Enthusiastic Eating

To overcome passionate eating, you have to retune your body to begin gaining from its prompts. It is an outlook change, not an eating routine, or a handy solution. In any case, when you build a training, it can give long haul results and advantages that outperform any eating regimen. As indicated by Gill, there are four key territories to deal with: passionate mindfulness, beating yearnings, taking care of segment control, and settling on sound decisions. Only in this case, it is possible to achieve a balanced ratio of nutrients and indispensable nutrition factors, to ensure not only a high level of digestion and absorption of nutrients but also their transportation to tissues and cells, their complete assimilation at the cell level. Synthetic nutrition ensures proper growth and formation of the body, contributes to maintaining health, high efficiency and prolonging life.

Equally important is the health and the environment. Human intervention in the regulation of natural processes does not always bring the desired positive results.

Violation of at least one of the natural components "leads, due to the interconnections between them, to restructuring the existing structure of natural-territorial components." Pollution of the surface of the land, hydrosphere, atmosphere and the oceans, in turn, affects the state of human health, the effect of the "ozone hole" affects the formation of malignant tumors, air pollution affects the state of the respiratory tract, and water pollution affects the digestion, dramatically worsens the general condition human health, reduces life expectancy. However, the health obtained from nature depends on parents only by 5%, and by 50% on the conditions surrounding us. In addition, it is necessary to take into account another objective factor of health effects - heredity. Biological rhythms affect our health. One of the most critical features of the processes taking place in a living organism is their rhythmic nature. Currently, it has been established that over three hundred processes occurring in the human body the optimal motor mode is the most critical condition for a healthy lifestyle. It is based on systematic exercises in physical exercises and sports, which effectively solve the tasks of strengthening the health and development of the physical abilities of youth, maintaining health and motor skills, and strengthening the prevention of adverse age-related changes. At the same time, material culture and sport act as the most important means of education. For effective healing and disease prevention, it is necessary to train and improve, first of all, the most valuable quality - endurance combined with hardening and other components of a healthy lifestyle, which will provide the growing body with a reliable shield against many diseases. Another critical element of a healthy lifestyle is personal hygiene. Personal hygiene includes a balanced daily regimen, body care, health of clothes and shoes. Of particular importance is the daily routine. With proper and strict adherence to it, a precise rhythm of the functioning of the body is produced. And this, in turn, creates the best conditions for work and recovery. Unequal conditions of life, work and life, individual differences of people do not allow recommending one variant of the daily regimen for all. However, its main provisions should be respected by all: "the implementation of various activities at a strictly defined time, the correct alternation of work and rest, regular nutrition. Particular attention should be paid to sleep - the primary and irreplaceable form of relaxation. Constant lack of sleep is dangerous because it can cause depletion of the nervous system, weakening the body's defenses, decreased performance, and poor health.

Enthusiastic Mindfulness

Know about any intense subject matters that affect your relationship with food and eating when you eat for different reasons than certified physical yearning. If you find that passionate variables drive your craving to eat, for example, eating for comfort because of stress, forlornness, and so on, what you need to do is fabricate another relationship with food, one that depends on a conscious choice to eat just when you're eager which will prompt more profitable purposeful food decisions. He regimen has not only healing but also educational value. Strict adherence to it brings up such qualities as discipline, accuracy, organization, determination. The mode allows a person to rationally use every hour, every minute of his time, which dramatically expands the possibility of a versatile and meaningful life. Each person should develop a regime based on the specific conditions of his life. Protecting one's own health is the immediate responsibility of everyone; he is not entitled to transfer it to others. After all, it often happens that a person with the wrong way of life, bad habits, physical inactivity, overeating brings himself to a catastrophic state by the age of 20-30 and only then remembers medicine. No matter how perfect cure is, it cannot save everyone from all diseases. Man is the creator of his own health, for which he must fight. From an early age, it is necessary to lead an active lifestyle, to harden, engage in physical education and sports, observe the rules of personal hygiene, and achieve reasonable harmony of health inconsistent ways. Health is the first and most important human need, which determines his ability to work and ensures the harmonious development of the individual. It is the most critical prerequisite for knowledge of the world, for self-affirmation and human happiness. Active long life is an essential component of the human factor.

Healthy lifestyle (HLS) is a lifestyle based on the principles of morality, rationally organized, active, labour, tempering and, at the same time, protecting from adverse environmental influences, allowing to maintain moral, mental and physical health until old age. There are three types of health: physical, mental and moral (social): - Physical fitness is the natural state of the body, due to the normal functioning of all its organs and systems. If all organs and systems work well, then the whole human body (self- regulating system) functions and develops correctly. - Mental health depends on the state of the brain, and it is characterized by the level and quality of thinking, the development of attention and memory, the degree of emotional stability, the development of volitional attributes. - Good health is determined by those ethical principles that are the basis of a person's social life, i.e. life in a particular human society. The hallmarks of human moral health are, first of all, a conscious attitude to work, mastery of cultural treasures, active rejection of mores and habits that contradict a usual way of life. A physically and mentally healthy person can be a good freak if he neglects ethical standards.

Those occasions when we're surrendering to the enticements of sugar, the psyche is in protection mode when we're sheltered. That is the reason we're naturally constrained to go after bites or indulge. Our mind has discovered that sweet tidbits or that sentiment of being overfull liken to "health." Beating food enslavement requires something more than self-discipline. Indeed, you heard that right; you Needn't bother with determination to defeat food compulsion. You need to retrain your subconscious mind-brain to help and discharge those programmed yearnings. That is the reason spellbinding for food fixation can be so useful.

Spellbinding permits us to get to the inner mind. What's more, when we talk straightforwardly to the psyche, we can start discharging unfortunate propensities and retraining our inner soul to be a supporter. It's in reality significantly more straightforward than it sounds. We can talk legitimately to it and feed it positive confirmations and new data to utilize. Because of trance, we can reprogram our awareness.

How Is The Sleeve Gastrectomy Performed?

Most of LSG's performed today are finished laparoscopically. During the LSG, around 75 percent of the stomach is expelled, leaving a tight gastric cylinder or "sleeve." No digestive organs are evacuated or skirted during the method, and it takes around one to two hours to finish. When contrasted with the gastric detour, the LSG can offer a shorter employable time that can be a preferred position for patients with extreme heart or lung ailment. The LSG technique enormously decreases the size of the stomach and restrains the measure of food that can be eaten at once. It doesn't cause diminished retention of supplements or sidestep the digestion tracts. After this medical procedure, patients feel full in the wake of eating exceptionally modest quantities of food. LSG may likewise cause a loss in craving. By and large, by year three, sleeve patients lost around 21 percent of their all-out body (weight at the time of technique). In a 350 pound individual, this would mean a 74- pound weight loss.

Complexities

LSG has been utilized effectively for a wide range of kinds of people influenced by extreme stoutness. Since it is a generally new technique, there is no information in regards to weight loss or weight-recover past three years. The danger of death from LSG is 0.2 percent (2 of every 1000) inside 30 days after a medical procedure. The threat of significant post-employable inconveniences after LSG is 5-10 percent, not precisely the hazard related to gastric detour. This is basically because the small digestive tract isn't partitioned and reconnected during LSG when contrasted with the detour techniques. This lower chance and shorter employable time is the fundamental purpose behind use as an organizing technique for high-hazard patients. Entanglements that can happen after LSG include: a break from the sleeve that can bring about a disease or ulcer, profound venous apoplexy (blood clump) or pneumonic embolism, and narrowing of the envelope (injury) requiring endoscopic widening and dying. Significant intricacies requiring re-activity are phenomenal after sleeve gastrectomy and happen in under 5 percent of patients. LSG is a bariatric medical procedure strategy that can prompt critical weight loss. Similarly, as with any bariatric medical procedure strategy, the best outcomes are accomplished when the medical procedure is joined with a multi-disciplinary program that centers around the way of life and social changes.

For Instance

you usually get in shape all the more rapidly after a gastric detour or sleeve gastrectomy than after gastric banding more individuals will, in general, accomplish critical weight loss with a gastric detour or sleeve gastrectomy than with a gastric band the danger of genuine medical procedure entanglements is commonly more significant for a gastric detour or sleeve gastrectomy gastric groups are removable, so the activity can be turned around if it causes substantial issues In case you're thinking about weight loss medical procedure, converse with your specialist about the various methods to conclude which is best for you. Appraisal before weight loss medical procedure Before you can have a weight loss medical procedure, you'll be alluded to an expert center for an appraisal to check if the activity is appropriate.

This May Include Checking Your

- Physical health – utilizing blood tests, X-beams and sweeps

- Diet and eating designs

- Mental health

For example, getting some information about your desires for a medical procedure, and whether you have any emotional health conditions; this is to evaluate on the off chance that you'll have the option to adapt to the drawn- out way of life changes required after weight loss medical procedure You might be encouraged to have a calorie-controlled eating routine in the prior week's medical system to help decrease the size of your liver. This can make the therapeutic procedure more straightforward and more secure. Dynamic Foundation Laparoscopic adjustable gastric banding (LAGB) is the third most well-known bariatric technique around the world. Different creators present irresolute long haul follows up results.

Techniques

We amended records of the patients who experienced LAGB somewhere in the range of 2003 and 2006 alongside the history of additional registration. Patients with obsolete subtleties were followed by the national medical coverage database and online networking (Facebook). An online study was sent. The patients who didn't have their band evacuated were remembered for this investigation. We determined the percent absolute weight loss (%TWL) and percent overabundance weight loss (%EWL), alongside changes in weight list (Triangle BMI).

Palatable weight loss was set at >50% EWL (for BMI = 25 kg/m2). Since eight patients put on weight, we chose to incorporate negative estimations of %TWL, %EWL, and Triangle BMI.

Results

One hundred seven patients experienced LAGB from 2003 to 2006. The mean follow-up time was 11.2 (±1.2) years. Eleven percent of patients were lost to development (n = 12). There was one perioperative passing. Fifty-four of the patients (n = 57) had their band expelled. Despite everything, thirty-

seven patients have the band (39%) and were remembered for the investigation. Twelve patients accomplished %EWL > half (32%). Thirty-two patients, despite everything, experience the ill effects of weight, with a BMI of more than 30 kg/m2. Eight patients (22%) put on extra weight. Patients with

%EWL > half experienced less gastroesophageal reflux infection manifestations than those with EWL < half (p < 0.05).

Ends

Out of 107 cases, just 11.2% of patients with a gastric band (n = 12) accomplished good %EWL. Twenty–two percent of patients recaptured their weight or even surpassed it. In general, outcomes recommend that LAGB isn't a powerful bariatric system in long haul perception.

Results

CONCLUSION

Thank you for reading all this book!

You can grasp why weight loss has been an issue previously and show up at a spot where you're mentally masterminded to hold fast to a health improvement plan and get to (and keep) your ideal weight. You'll, in like manner, watch the mind obstructs that keep you from the positive turn of events, for instance, fears created from your childhood that are appearing in self-damage.

You have already taken a step towards your improvement.

Best wishes!

CPSIA information can be obtained
at www.ICGtesting.com
Printed in the USA
BVHW041528210321
602995BV00022B/51